UNDERSTANDING DISORDERS



# WHAT ARE EATING DISORDERS?

by Tammy Gagne

BrightPoint Press

San Diego, CA

BrightPoint Press


an imprint of ReferencePoint Press, Inc.
Printed in the United States

For more information, contact:
BrightPoint Press
PO Box 27779
San Diego, CA 92198
www.BrightPointPress.com



Content Consultant: Kyle De Young, PhD, Fellow of the Academy for Eating Disorders, Associate Professor of Psychology, University of Wyoming

LIBRARY OF CONGRESS CATALOGING-IN-PUBLICATION DATA

Names: Gagne, Tammy, author.
Title: What are eating disorders? / by Tammy Gagne.
Description: San Diego, CA : BrightPoint Press, [2023] | Series: Understanding disorders | Includes bibliographical references and index. | Audience: Grades 10-12
Identifiers: LCCN 2022003705 (print) | LCCN 2022003706 (eBook) | ISBN 9781678204464 (hardcover) | ISBN 9781678204471 (eBook)
Subjects: LCSH: Eating disorders--Juvenile literature. | Eating disorders--Treatment--Juvenile literature.
Classification: LCC RC552.E18 G34 2023 (print) | LCC RC552.E18 (eBook) | DDC 616.85/26--dc23/eng/20220203
LC record available at https://lccn.loc.gov/2022003705
LC eBook record available at https://lccn.loc.gov/2022003706

# CONTENTS

# AT A GLANCE

- Eating disorders affect about 28.8 million people in the United States. These disorders affect physical and mental health.
- Many factors can increase the risk of developing an eating disorder. Certain genes and personality types are risk factors. Stress also plays a role.
- People with anorexia nervosa severely limit the amount of food they eat. This leads to an unhealthy amount of weight loss that can harm physical health.
- People with bulimia nervosa binge eat. They also purge, or do behaviors to get rid of calories. Vomiting and taking laxatives are purging behaviors.
- Binge eating is the main symptom of binge eating disorder. People with this disorder eat large amounts of food in a short period of time.

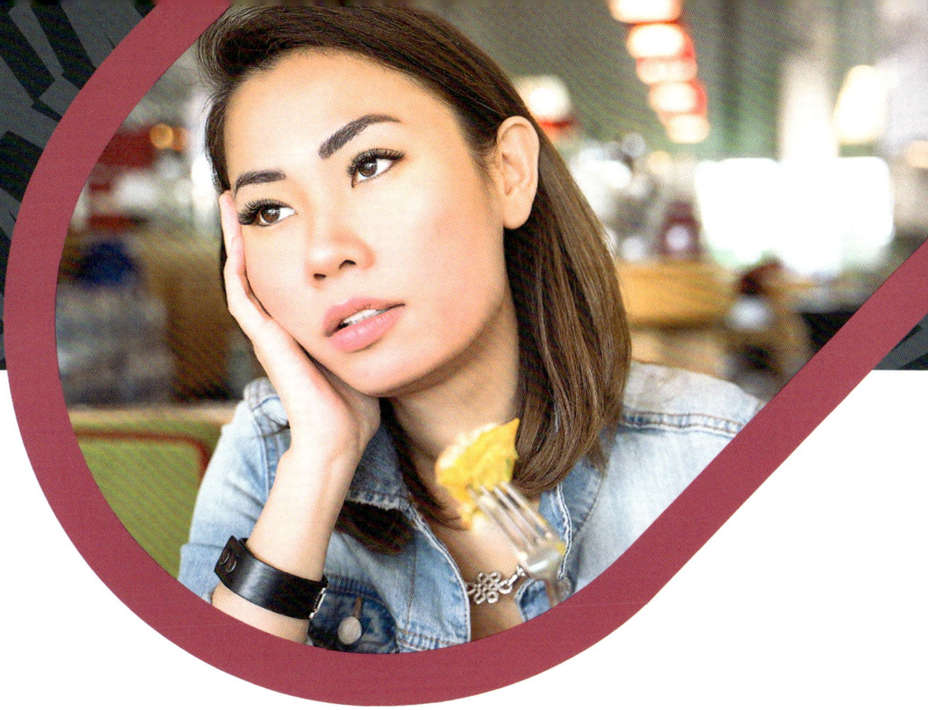

- Anybody can develop an eating disorder. Most research on eating disorders has focused on white females. This can make it difficult for men or people of color to get a diagnosis.
- Stigma can make it difficult for people with eating disorders to seek treatment.
- Eating disorders are treatable. Many people with eating disorders have improved with psychotherapy and nutrition plans. Some eating disorders can be treated with medicine.

# HELPING A FRIEND

Clara made sure they were alone before saying anything. She had followed Emily to the ladies' room at the pizza place. The rest of their basketball team was busy celebrating their latest win. Clara was nervous about how Emily would react. But she knew she was doing the right thing.

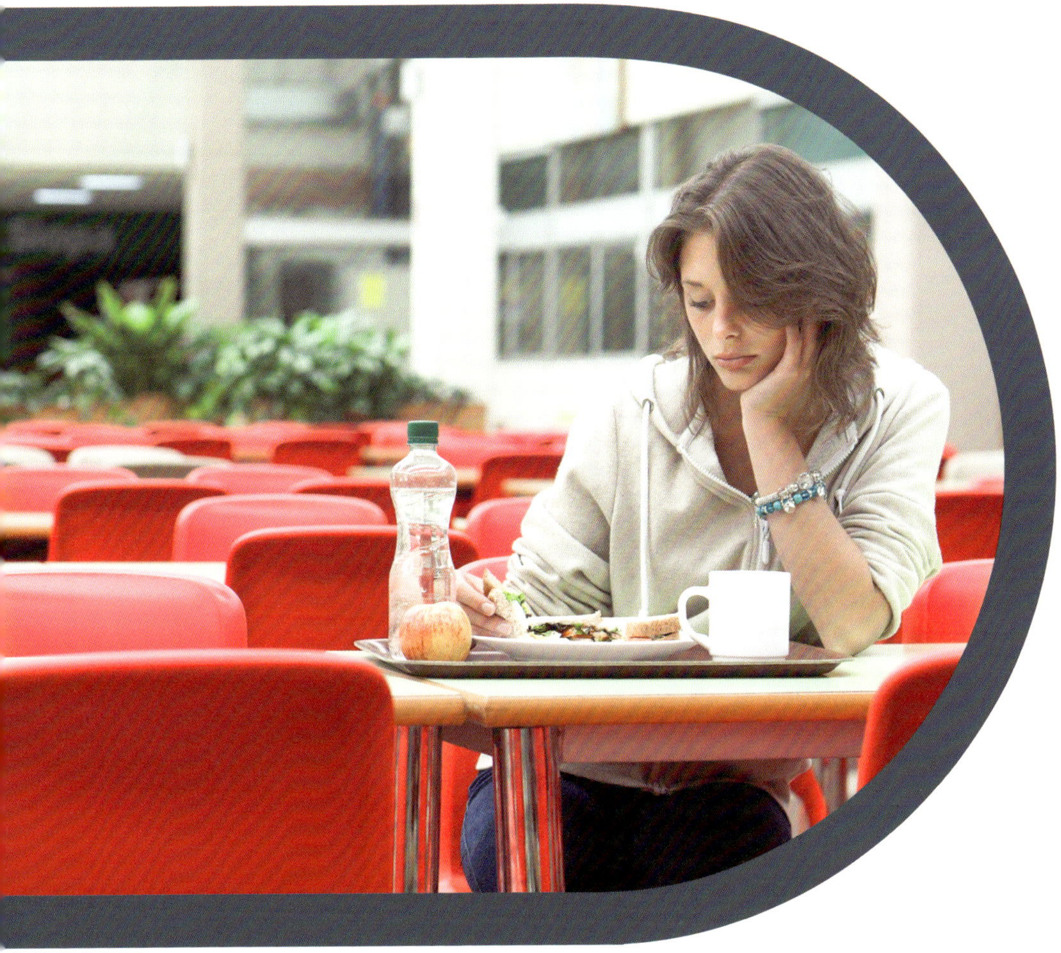

*Having an eating disorder can make it difficult to eat in front of others.*

Clara saw Emily's knees in front of the toilet in the last stall. She heard Emily vomiting. Emily stood as Clara approached. "I'm fine," Emily insisted.

"No, you're not," Clara said. "And I understand. Last year I was diagnosed with bulimia."

"What is that?" Emily asked.

"It's a disease. Only a mental health professional can diagnose it. But making yourself throw up is one of the symptoms."

"I feel so much pressure to be thin," Emily admitted.

"I get it," Clara reassured her. "First, you just want to be able to eat like everyone else. Then when you do, you feel guilty. So you think that you can get rid of all the **calories** you just ate. You think it's a

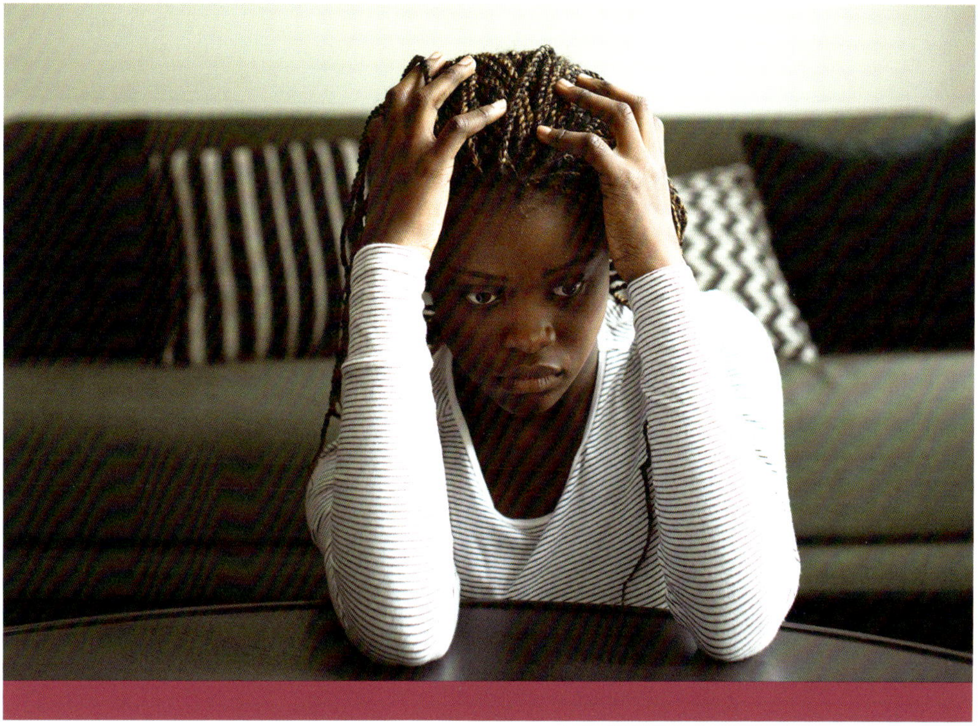

***Eating disorders can have a serious effect on physical and mental health.***

one-time thing. But then it happens again. Before you know it, it becomes a habit. You can't control it. But it's hurting you."

Emily didn't respond or come out of the stall. Clara continued. "You should tell your parents."

"How do I tell them?" Emily asked. "They won't understand. They'll think I'm crazy."

"My parents were shocked," Clara admitted. "But they got me the help I needed. I can go with you to talk to your parents if you want. What matters is that you get help. I see a therapist about my bulimia. It has made a big difference."

## WHAT ARE EATING DISORDERS?

There are several types of eating disorders. These mental illnesses affect eating habits. People with eating disorders feel distress about their eating behaviors.

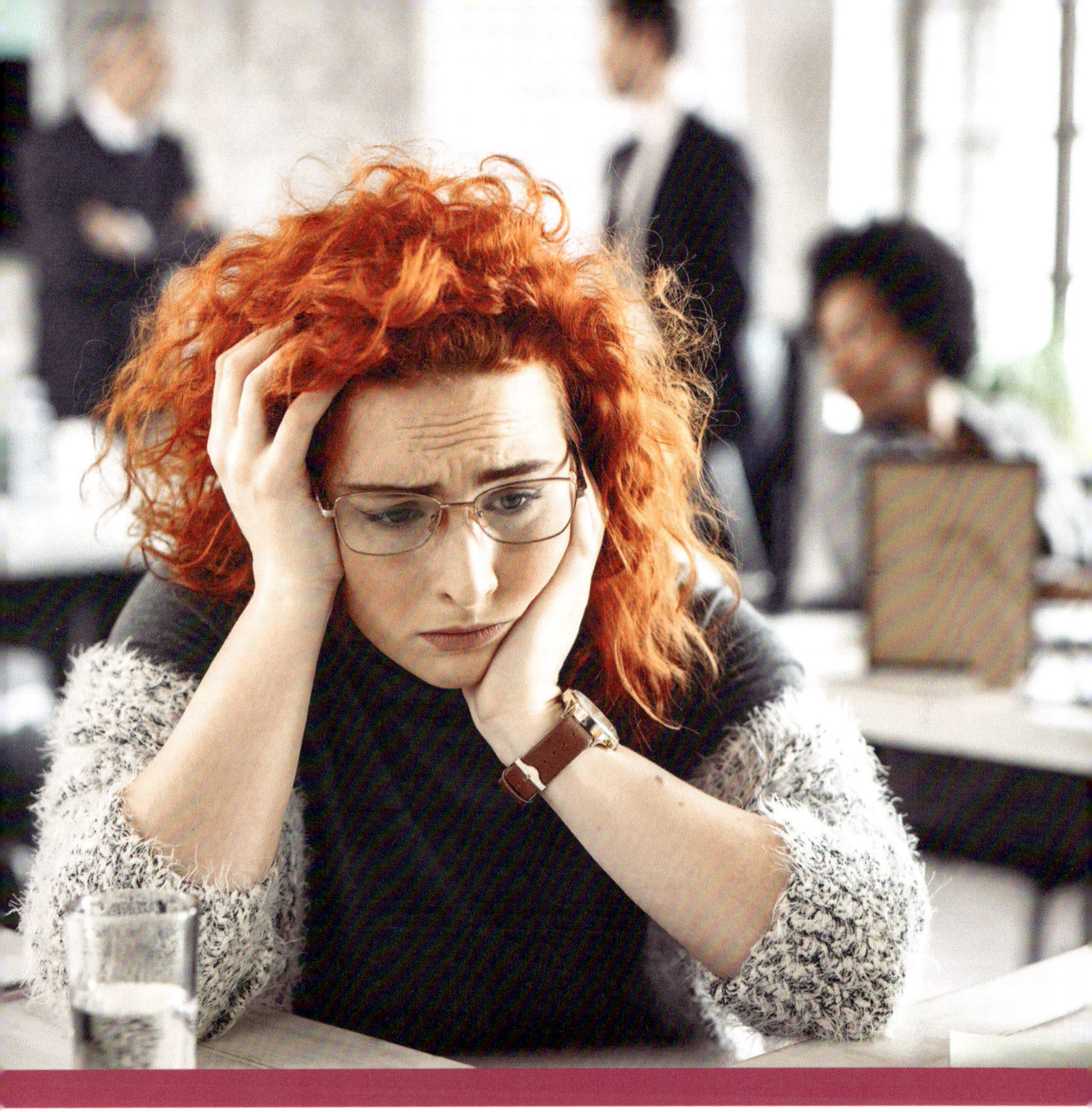

***Anxiety can worsen the eating habits of someone who has an eating disorder.***

Their eating habits harm their physical and mental health.

People with anorexia nervosa severely limit their food intake. They have an intense fear of gaining weight. Bulimia nervosa is another eating disorder. People with bulimia also fear weight gain. They may diet excessively. They may try to get rid of the food they have eaten by vomiting. Binge eating is another sign of bulimia. People may eat large amounts of food in a short time. This behavior is also seen in binge eating disorder. Other types of disordered eating also exist. Each eating disorder has its own set of symptoms.

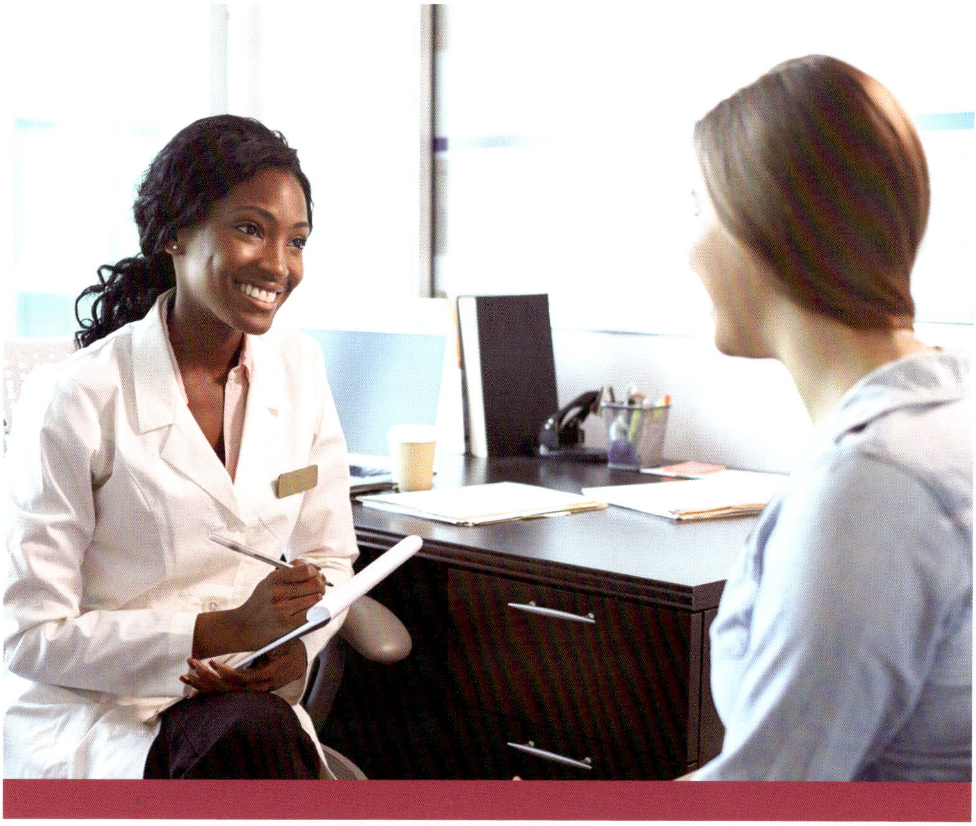

***A nutritionist can help someone with an eating disorder establish a healthy diet.***

Fighting an eating disorder isn't easy. But treatment is possible. With treatment, many people with eating disorders live healthy lives.

CHAPTER ONE

# THE HISTORY OF EATING DISORDERS

Disordered eating has existed for centuries. Extreme **fasting** was part of religious rituals in ancient times. Fasting was a way to become more spiritual. This behavior continued through the Middle Ages. It sometimes led to death. Saint Catherine of Siena died at the age of

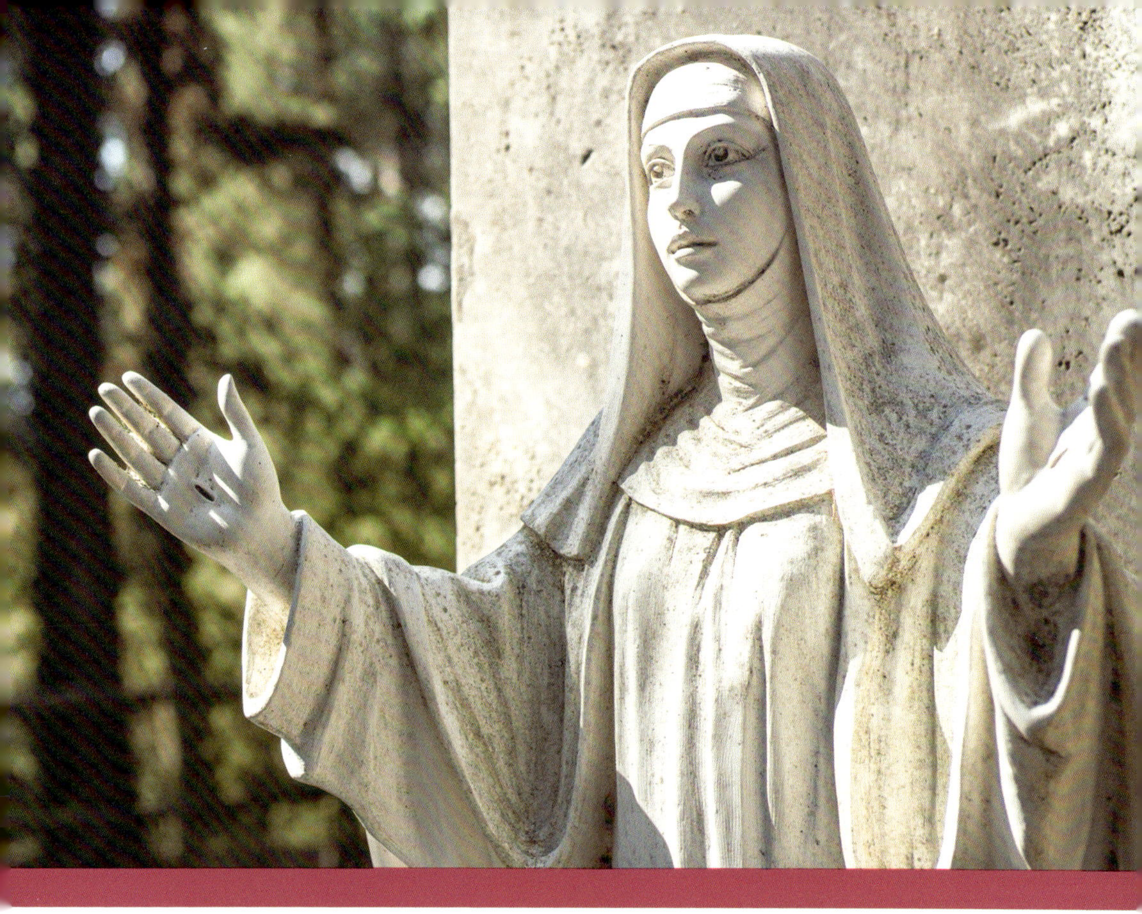

***Saint Catherine of Siena practiced extreme fasting. Some doctors today believe that this was a sign of an eating disorder.***

thirty-three in 1380. She did not eat for long periods of time. This may have led to her early death.

Other saints of this era also practiced fasting. These saints are often honored

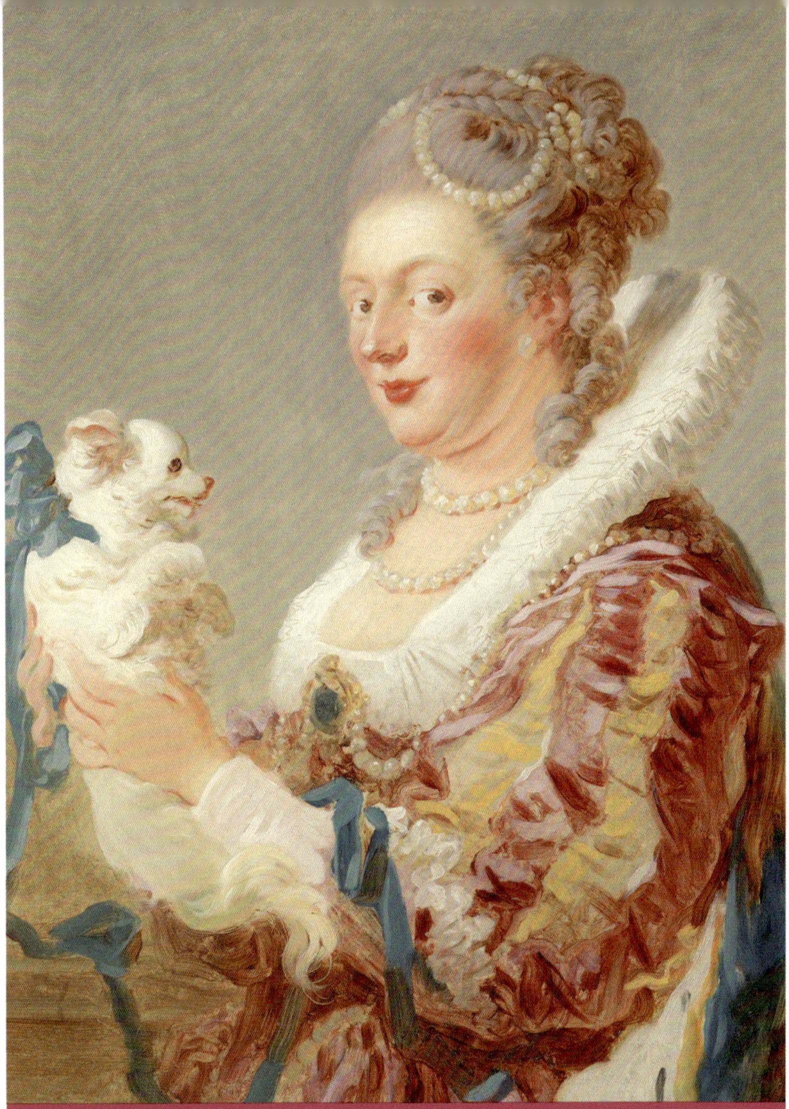

***Historically, excess body weight was seen as a symbol of wealth.***

for their strong faith. But some doctors believe that mental health issues may have also played a role in their extreme fasting.

Dr. James Greenblatt is a **psychiatrist**. He pointed out, "We can recognize from the lives of these [individuals] familiar symptoms: depression, anxiety, obsessive thoughts, and **compulsive** behaviors."[1] These symptoms may have caused fasting to become out of control. Fasting began to have a severe effect on their physical health.

Bulimia nervosa is an eating disorder. Signs of this disorder have been traced back to the Middle Ages. Some people of this time vomited to treat certain diseases. Forcing oneself to vomit can be a sign of bulimia.

## LEARNING MORE ABOUT EATING DISORDERS

In 1689, English doctor Richard Morton wrote about a condition. He called it wasting disease. He described two teenage patients. One was female. The other was male. Both experienced extreme weight loss. This weight loss was harmful to their health. In 1873, English doctor Sir William Gull named the disorder anorexia nervosa. He was the first to do so. Anorexia nervosa means "nervous loss of appetite." Patients with anorexia were extremely underweight. Gull also noticed that they were anxious.

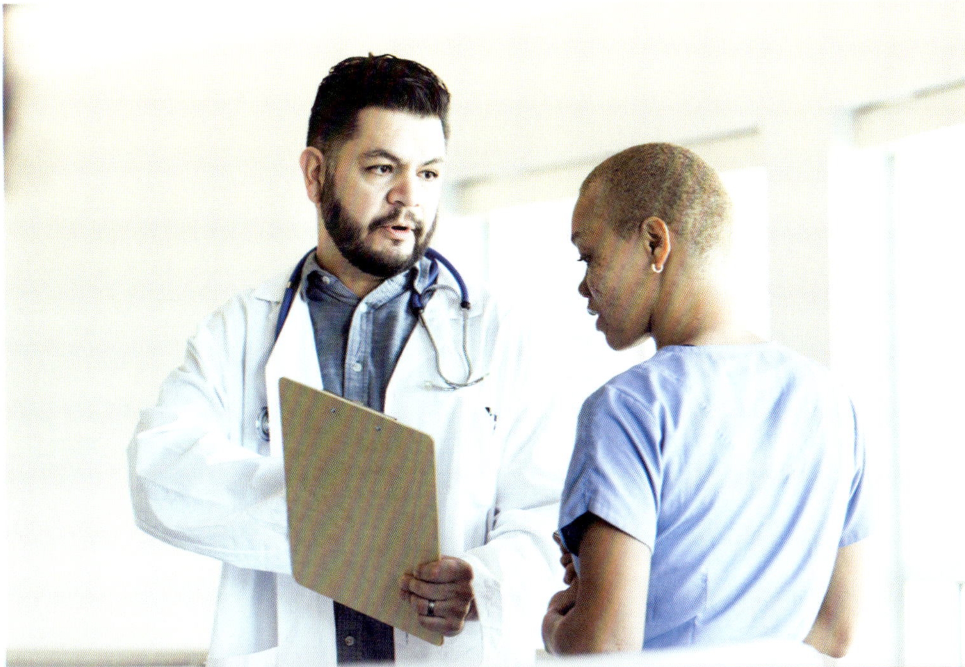

***Doctors continue to learn more about eating disorders.***

The medical community began to see anorexia as a mental illness around this time.

Doctors use the *Diagnostic and Statistical Manual of Mental Disorders* (*DSM*) to diagnose mental illnesses. Anorexia nervosa was the only named eating disorder for many years. This changed in 1979. That year, bulimia nervosa was first discussed as its own condition. Before then it was seen as a form of anorexia. Bulimia was added to the third edition of the *DSM* the following year. The *DSM-III* was also the

### FEEDING DISORDERS

The *DSM-IV* described childhood feeding disorders. Some children avoided many types of food. Others often ate items that were not food, such as dirt or paper. But doctors realized that these eating behaviors were also present in teens and adults. The *DSM-5* grouped eating and feeding disorders together. It also removed age limitations on these disorders.

first version to include a separate section on eating disorders.

New versions of the *DSM* are published as scientists learn more about mental health. Descriptions of eating disorders have changed over time. For example, the *DSM-IV* listed a new symptom. People with anorexia and bulimia may connect their self-worth with their weight. Binge eating disorder was added to the *DSM-5* as a new disorder.

## EARLY TREATMENTS

Doctors noticed that patients with anorexia made lower amounts of certain **hormones**.

The patients had low levels of pituitary hormones. Doctors believed that low levels of these hormones caused anorexia. They used pituitary hormones to treat patients with anorexia. They later learned that pituitary hormone levels did not cause anorexia. Instead, it was an effect of the disorder. Poor nutrition can lead to low levels of these hormones.

In 1947, a doctor named John M. Berkman studied anorexia nervosa. He worked with female patients at the Mayo Clinic in Minnesota. Berkman thought that a poor relationship with one's parents led

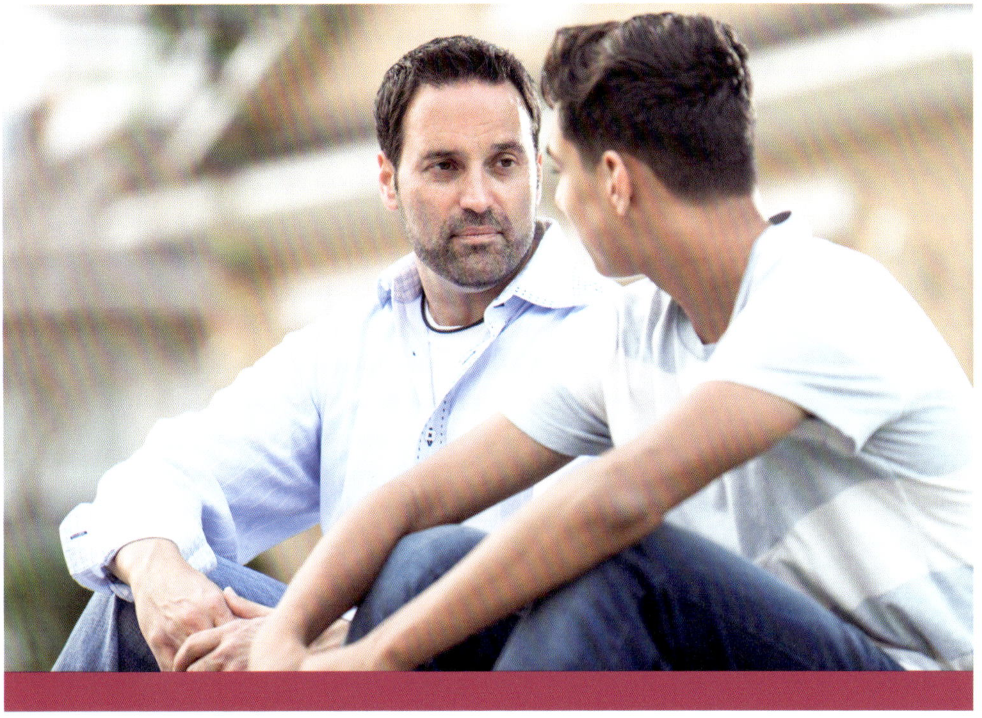

***Family support can help someone cope with an eating disorder.***

to the illness. This idea sparked a new treatment that involved removing children with anorexia from their parents' homes. This did not help patients. Instead, it was damaging for patients and their families. Modern treatments for eating disorders include family members. Research has shown that family-based treatment is effective.

## INCREASING AWARENESS

Hilde Bruch was an American psychiatrist. She raised public awareness about eating disorders in the 1970s. She studied people with these disorders. She wrote about her findings in a book. This led to greater awareness. Many people began seeking treatment for eating disorders.

Valerie Huntley developed an eating disorder when she was seventeen years old. She struggled with her illness for four years before getting treatment. Huntley is now a social worker. She helps other people who are suffering from eating disorders. She encourages them to get help. She said, "If I did not receive treatment, I would not be here today."[2]

### CHANGING ATTITUDES TOWARD BODY SHAPES

Excess body fat was once seen as a symbol of wealth. People in poverty struggled to get enough food. But the wealthiest individuals ate as much as they wanted. Modern culture has a different view of body weight. Many people want to appear thin. The rise of cities and technology has made food available to more people. People began to see thinness as a sign of self-control.

CHAPTER TWO

# NOTABLE EATING DISORDERS

Eating disorders affect about 28.8 million people in the United States. This is about 9 percent of the population. Some eating disorders are more common in females. But males suffer from them too. Many people believe **stereotypes** about eating disorders. They may think that all people with eating

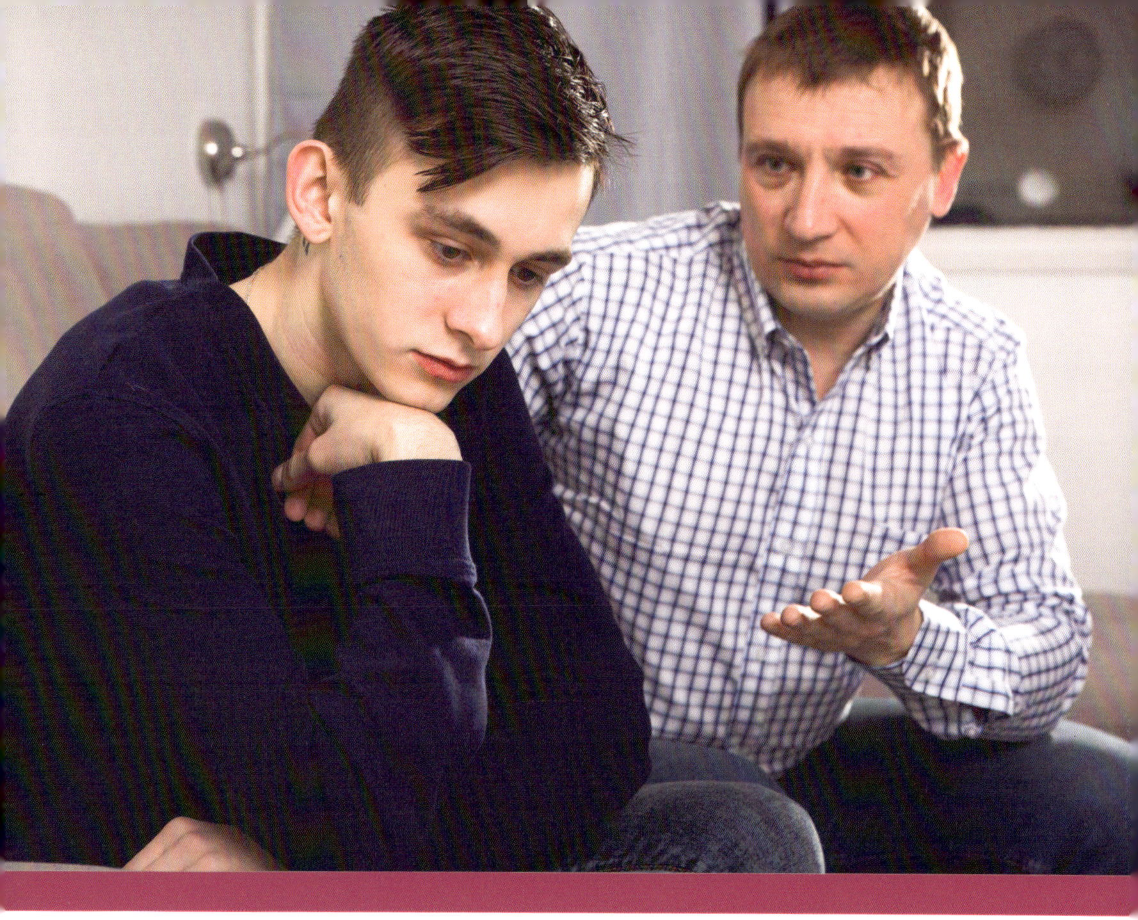

***It can be difficult for boys and men to receive an eating disorder diagnosis due to stereotypes.***

disorders are white females. Many studies focus on this part of the population.

Stereotypes can make it difficult for men to receive the right diagnoses. They may prevent men and boys from getting help.

Dr. Jason Nagata is a doctor and researcher at the University of California, San Francisco. He said, "A lot of boys and men go unrecognized, and they have delays in getting care."[3]

People of color also suffer from eating disorders. Black teens are 50 percent more likely than their white peers to suffer from bulimia. Hispanic people are also more likely

### A GLOBAL ISSUE

**Eating disorders have been diagnosed in most areas of the world. Japan, Pakistan, the United Kingdom, and the United States are just a few of the nations that have seen an increase in eating disorders in recent decades.**

## Rate of Eating Disorders Among Women of Different Races

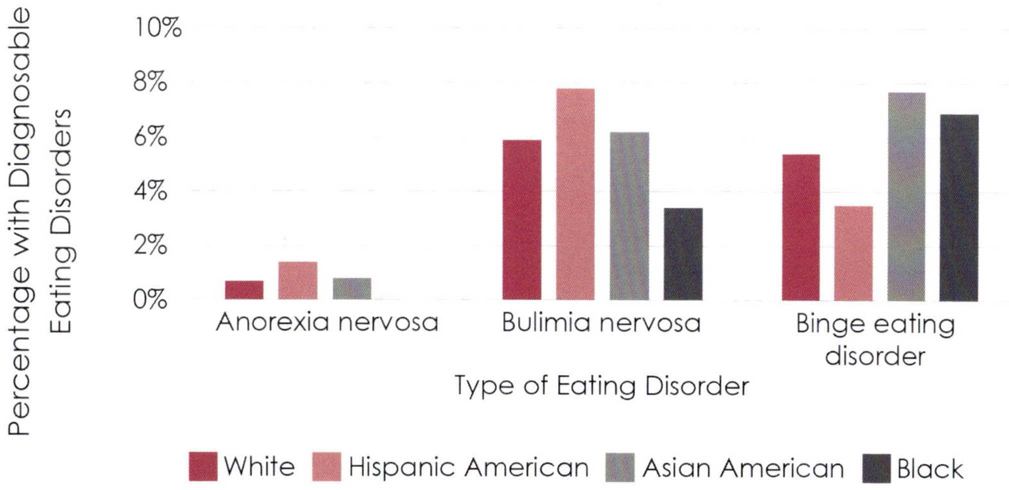


*Source: Zhen Hadassah Cheng et al., "Ethnic Differences in Eating Disorder Prevalence, Risk Factors, and Predictive Effects of Risk Factors Among Young Women,"* NCBI, *January 2019. www.ncbi.nlm.nih.gov.*

***A 2019 study looked at the rates of eating disorders in 848 white women, 141 Hispanic women, 130 Asian women, and 58 Black women.***

to suffer from this disorder. But doctors are less likely to ask people of color about eating behaviors. This can make it difficult for them to receive treatment.

## RISK FACTORS

Certain risk factors make it more likely to develop an eating disorder. One risk factor is family history. This is especially true for anorexia. People with a family history of this disorder are at high risk. They are eleven times more likely to develop the disorder than someone without this family history. Family history also influences bulimia.

Stress can lead to an eating disorder. Going to a new school can cause people to change their eating behaviors. Mental health conditions such as anxiety can also make an eating disorder more likely.

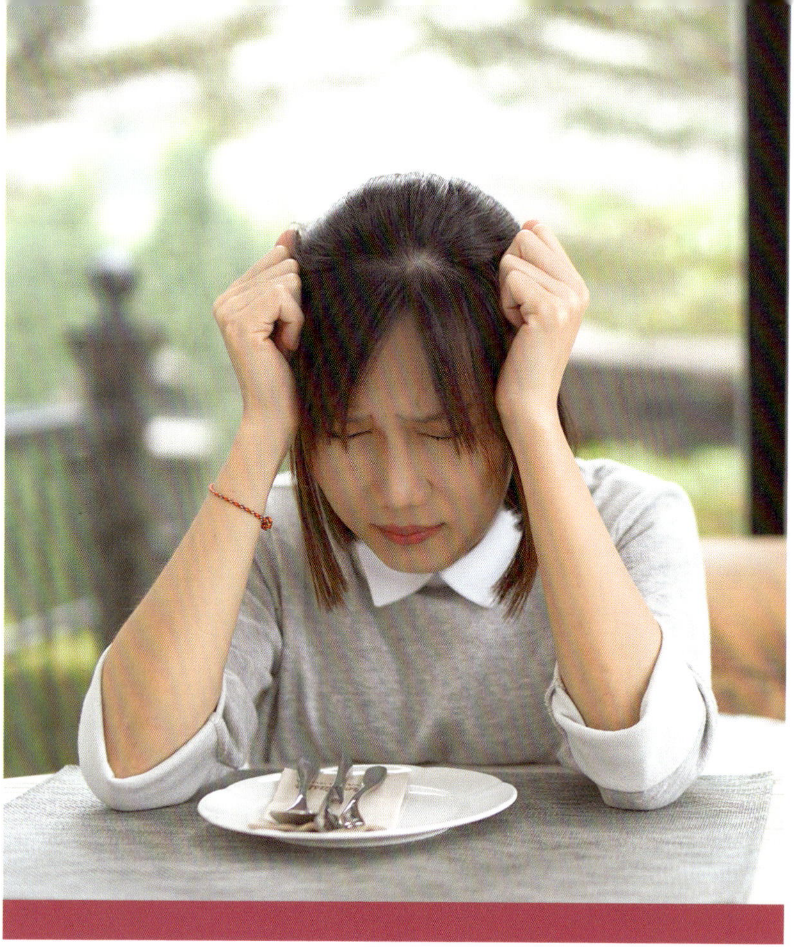

*Stress can cause a change in eating behaviors.*

Some people with eating disorders worry about being perfect. They may stop eating to punish themselves. Or they may believe that they must be thin to be perfect. This way of thinking is another risk factor.

## ANOREXIA NERVOSA

Anorexia nervosa is a well-known eating disorder. It affects less than 1 percent of the US population. Most people with anorexia are diagnosed as teens or young adults. But children and older adults can also develop anorexia.

People with anorexia strictly limit the amount of food they eat. They avoid foods that they consider to be fattening. Men typically need about 2,500 calories a day. Women should eat around 2,000 calories. The number of calories a person needs varies. Age and activity level influence

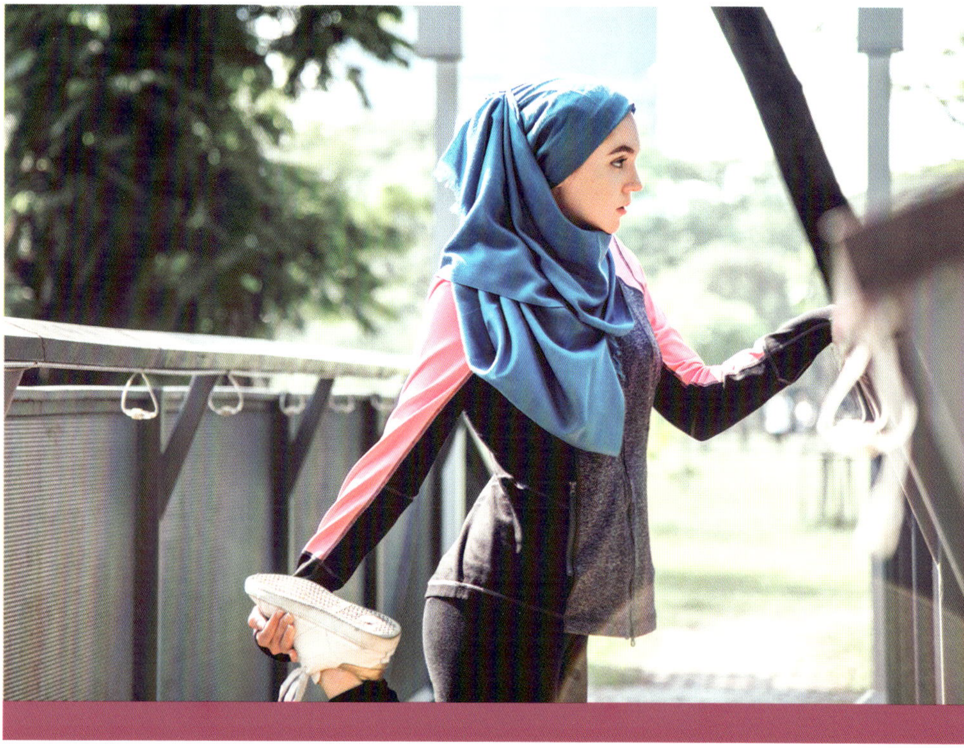

***Someone who exercises often needs more calories to stay healthy.***

this amount. Someone with anorexia may routinely eat less than 1,000 calories per day.

This behavior causes adults to become severely underweight. Children and teens with anorexia may not gain weight. There may be delays in developmental milestones such as puberty. The starvation puts a lot of stress on the body. Complications from anorexia can even lead to death.

People with anorexia have an intense fear of being overweight. They do not eat when

## MEDIA AND BODY IMAGE

**Studies have linked the media's focus on being thin with disordered eating. One study revealed that young girls who frequently read about fashion were twice as likely to go on diets as their peers. They were three times more likely to exercise to lose weight. Another study looked at diet habits of children. Some wanted to look like the people they see in media. These children had a higher risk of becoming constant dieters than peers without this desire.**

they are hungry. They diet obsessively. They may exercise to an extreme. Patients often feel anxious and depressed. They may not recognize how thin they have become. They may still believe they are overweight even when their weight loss is harmful to their health.

## BULIMIA NERVOSA

Bulimia nervosa is often diagnosed in the late teen years. But this eating disorder can affect people at any age. People with bulimia also fear becoming overweight. They try to limit their calorie intake. This may involve fasting or dieting. But people with

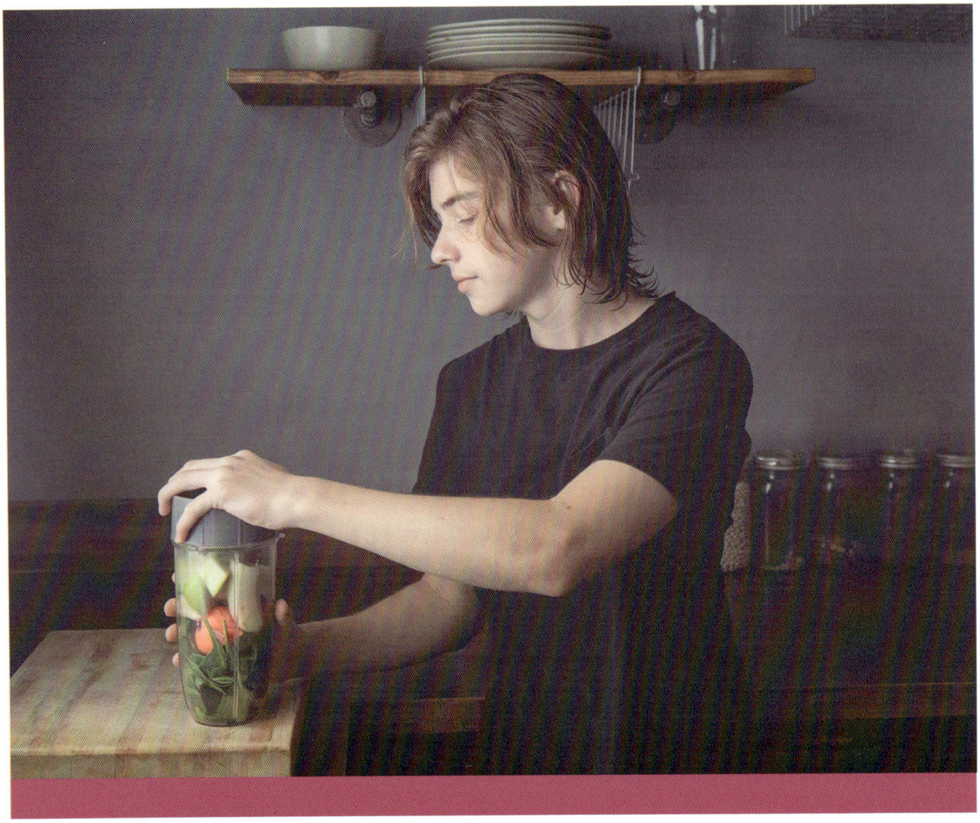

***Eating after exercise is important for the body's recovery.***

bulimia do not experience extreme weight loss. This disorder still has a severe impact on health. People with bulimia are often anxious. Their eating behaviors put a lot of stress on their bodies.

One sign of bulimia is binge eating. People with bulimia eat large amounts of food in short periods of time. They feel like they lose control when they binge. They feel as though they cannot stop bingeing.

Afterward they may feel guilty about the amount of food they have eaten. They try to get rid of the food in their bodies. This is called purging. There are many purging behaviors. Vomiting is common. People with bulimia may also use **laxatives**.

These behaviors are unhealthy. They are also not effective ways to lose weight. The body absorbs calories as soon as

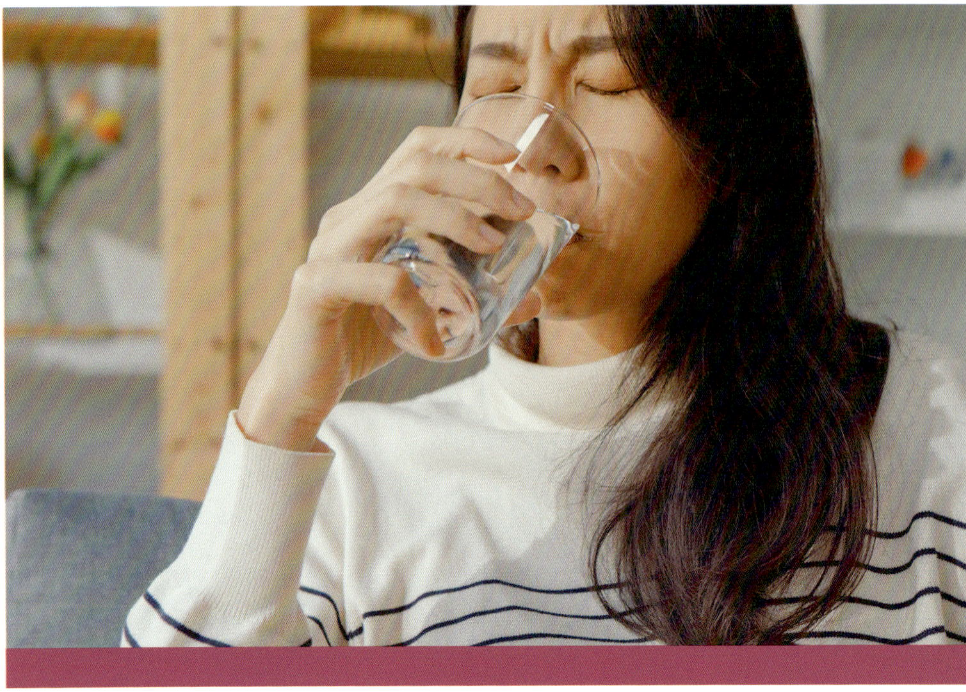

***Taking laxatives does not help a person lose weight. Abusing these drugs can harm a person's health.***

food is eaten. Vomiting gets rid of less than 50 percent of calories. Laxatives are even less effective. It is also difficult to lose weight through extreme diets. These diets cause the body to burn calories at a much slower rate.

People with bulimia may experience intense urges. This leads them to binge and purge. They may feel relieved after doing these things. But the relief is soon replaced with guilt and shame. People may try to control these negative feelings through their eating behaviors. This cycle of emotions can make it difficult to stop bingeing and purging. These eating behaviors must last for three months to receive a bulimia diagnosis. A person with this diagnosis engages in bingeing and purging an average of at least once a week during that time.

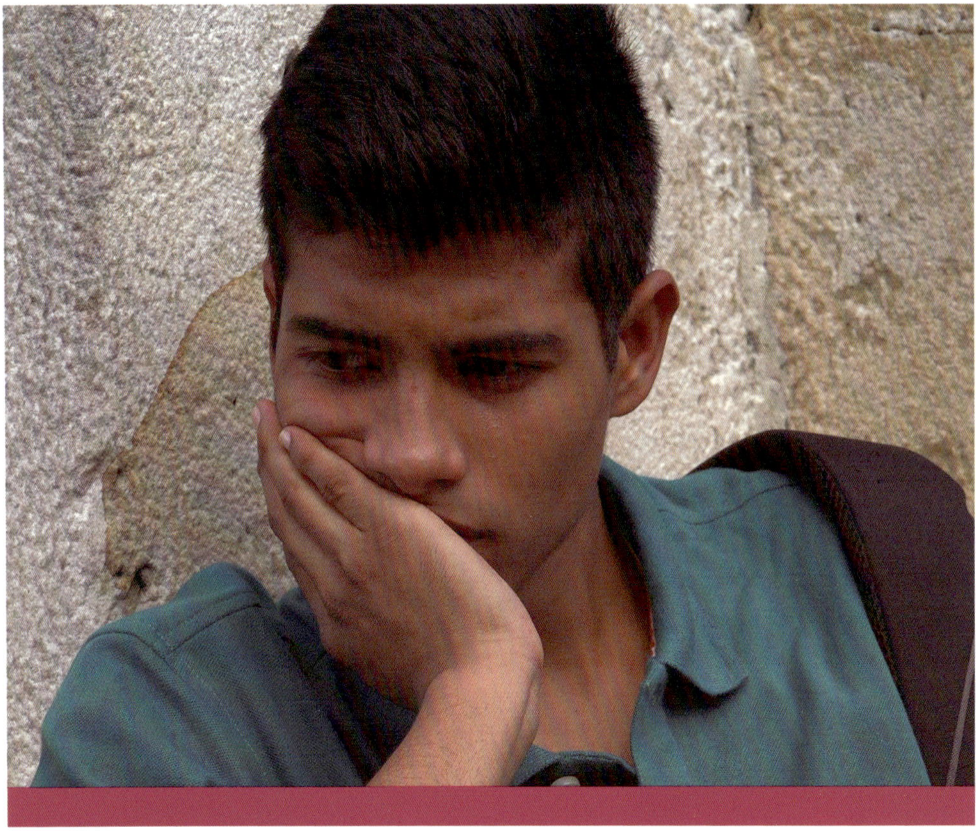

***Someone with an eating disorder may feel ashamed about his eating behaviors.***

## BINGE EATING DISORDER

Binge eating disorder is the most common eating disorder in the United States. More women are diagnosed with this disorder than men. But the difference is not as extreme as with anorexia or bulimia. Binge eating disorder is commonly diagnosed in young adults. This is later than what is seen in anorexia and bulimia.

People with binge eating disorder eat large amounts of food. But they do not purge. This can cause weight gain. But many people with this disorder are not overweight. People may eat rapidly during a binge. They may binge even when they are not hungry. Many people with this illness are ashamed of their eating behavior. They may not want to eat in front of others. They may feel guilty or disgusted after bingeing.

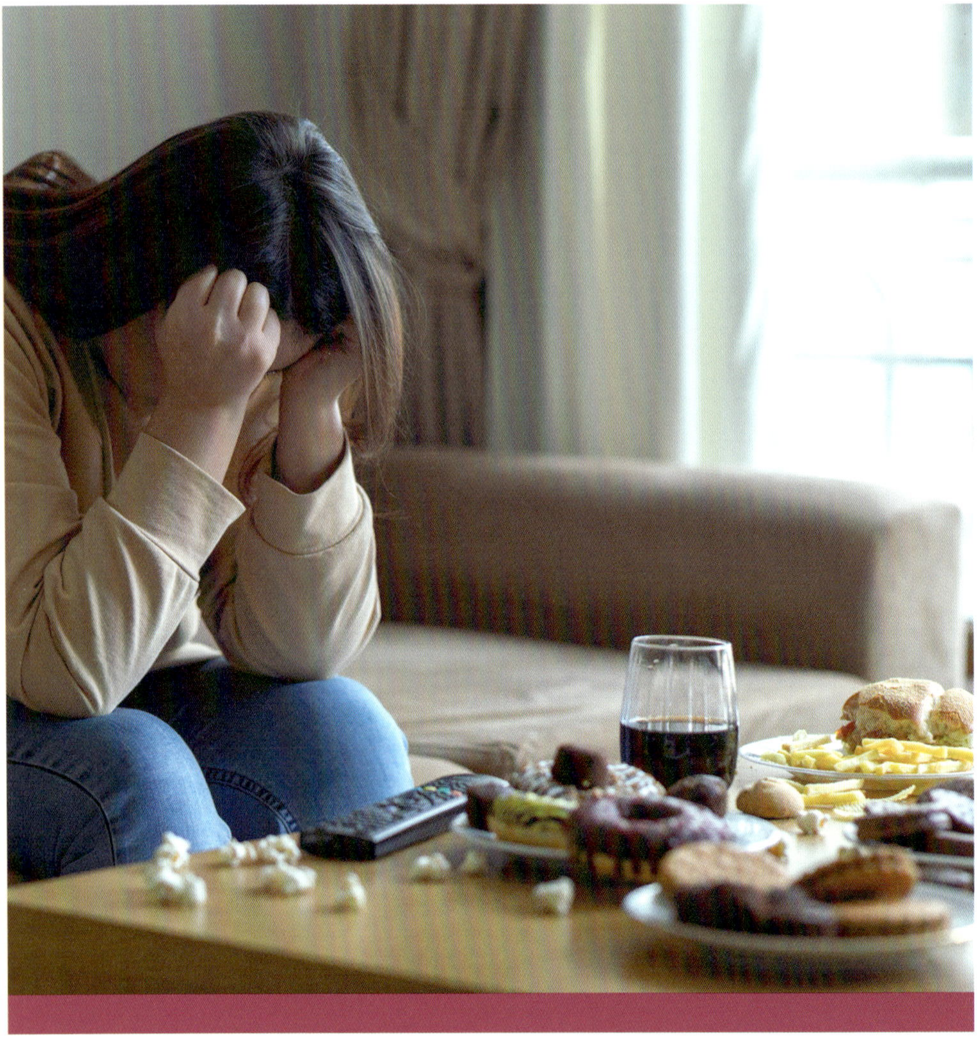

***Shame surrounding binge eating can cause people to withdraw from those close to them.***

Many factors can cause someone to binge eat. Stress is one factor. Certain foods may trigger binge eating. People with binge eating disorder know their behavior is unhealthy. But it is very difficult to stop a binge.

Sally Slater started binge eating when she was fifteen. Most people need about 2,000 calories a day. Sally sometimes ate 10,000 calories in one sitting. "It seems so simple to put the food down," she said, "but it's more complicated than that."[4]

## OTHER EATING DISORDERS

Avoidant/restrictive food intake disorder (ARFID) is another eating disorder. Some people mistake the disorder for picky eating. But people with ARFID avoid a wide variety of foods. Some people avoid foods because of their texture. Others have no interest in eating. They do not avoid food to lose weight. But food avoidance can lead to extreme weight loss. ARFID can lead to developmental delays in children and teens.

ARFID is more common in boys than girls. It tends to develop in childhood. But teens and adults may also have ARFID.

The *DSM* also includes information on other specified feeding or eating disorder (OSFED). Patients with OSFED have symptoms that are similar to those of other eating disorders. For example, people

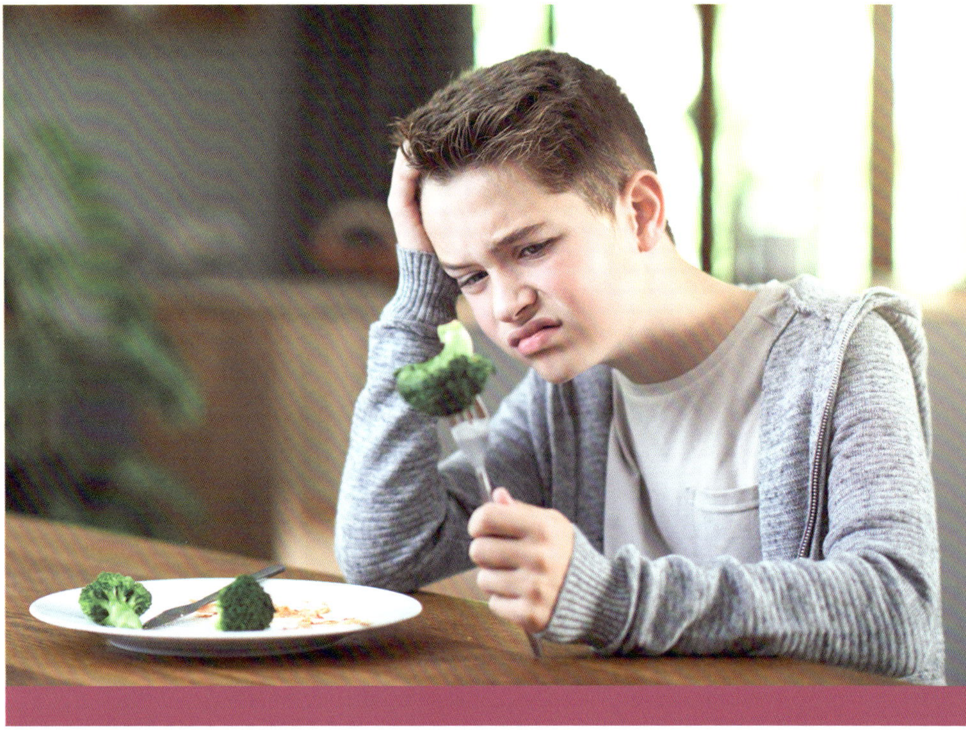

***Someone with ARFID may refuse to eat many types of food.***

with OSFED may have symptoms that are similar to bulimia symptoms. But they may not binge and purge often enough to be diagnosed with bulimia. Or they may purge without bingeing.

CHAPTER THREE

# EATING DISORDERS AND EVERYDAY LIFE

Living with an eating disorder isn't easy. Food is a big part of social gatherings. Friends may go to parties or restaurants together. Sport venues and movie theaters also provide food. People with eating disorders may avoid going to these places. They do not want to eat in front of their

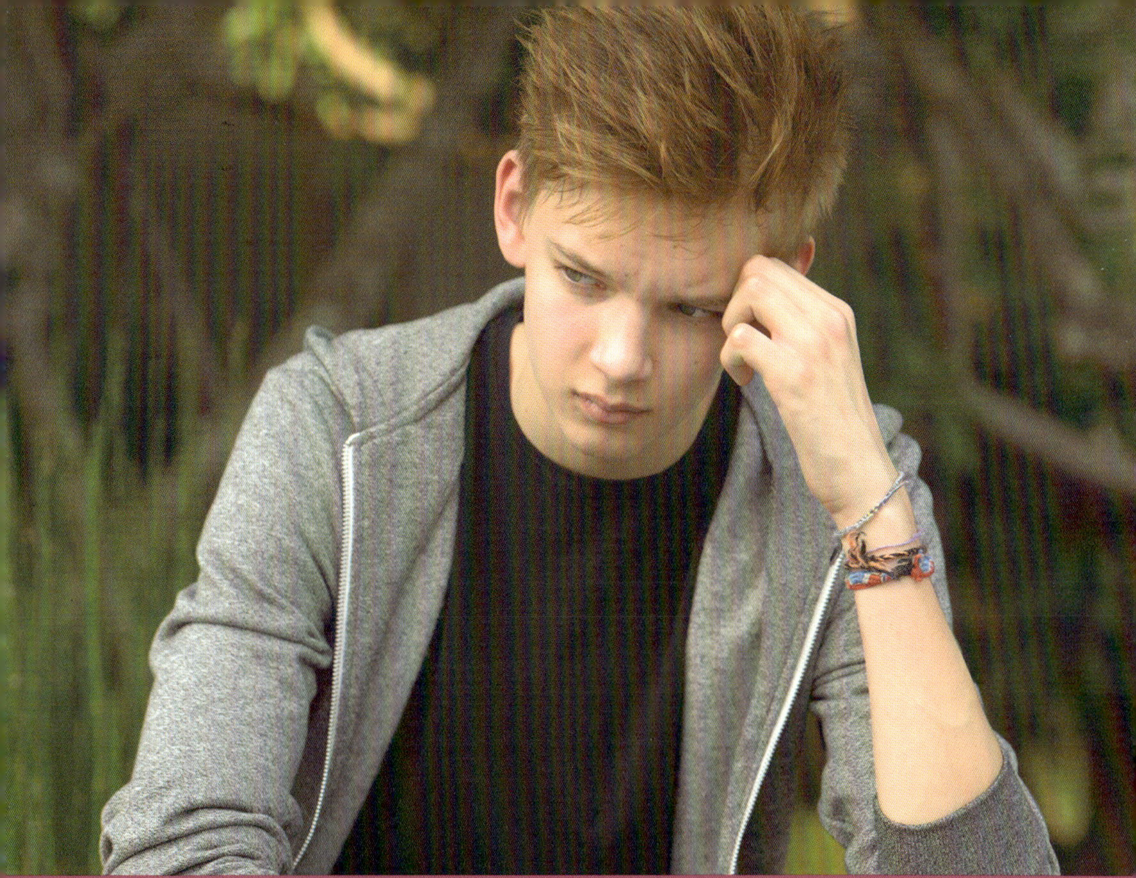

***An eating disorder can make it difficult to spend time with others.***

friends. Turning down invitations to hang out can damage relationships.

An eating disorder can also lead to a lack of energy. This can hurt relationships too. People with eating disorders may feel

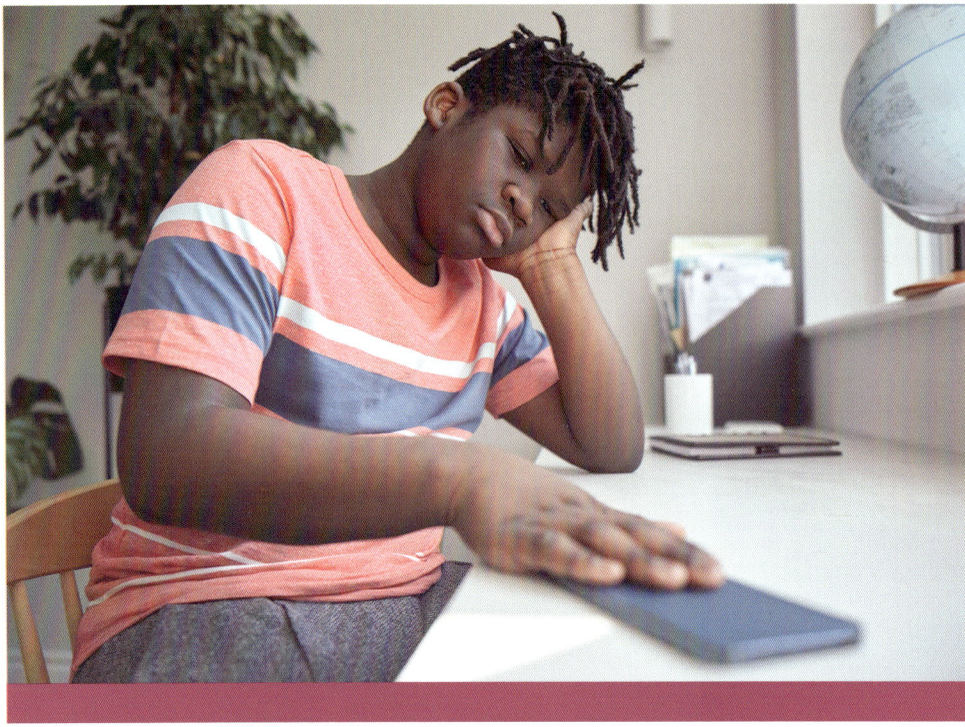

*Isolation can cause eating disorders to worsen.*

too tired to socialize. This was the case for Emily T. Troscianko. Her friendships suffered because of her anorexia. She wrote in her diary, "This food thing's beginning to scare me now; I'm always hungry, always tired. . . . I'm weighing myself every day now, I'm always thinking about food; how to avoid it or how to get it. But it's losing me my friends."[5]

## SELF-ESTEEM

People with eating disorders often suffer from low self-esteem. They may feel alone. They may believe they are not worthy of friendship. This can make it difficult to reach out for help. They might feel that they have no one to talk to about the disorder. These negative feelings can worsen the eating disorder.

People with eating disorders also face an increased risk for suicide. Suicide is the most common cause of death for people dealing with an eating disorder. Eating disorders can make a person feel hopeless and worthless. The person may mistakenly think there is no way out. Treatment is the best way to avoid these risks. Early treatment improves the chances of recovery.

## DEALING WITH STIGMA

There is a **stigma** surrounding eating disorders. Others may wrongly believe that people with eating disorders caused their illnesses. They may tell people with eating disorders to "just eat." They do not understand that recovery is not so simple.

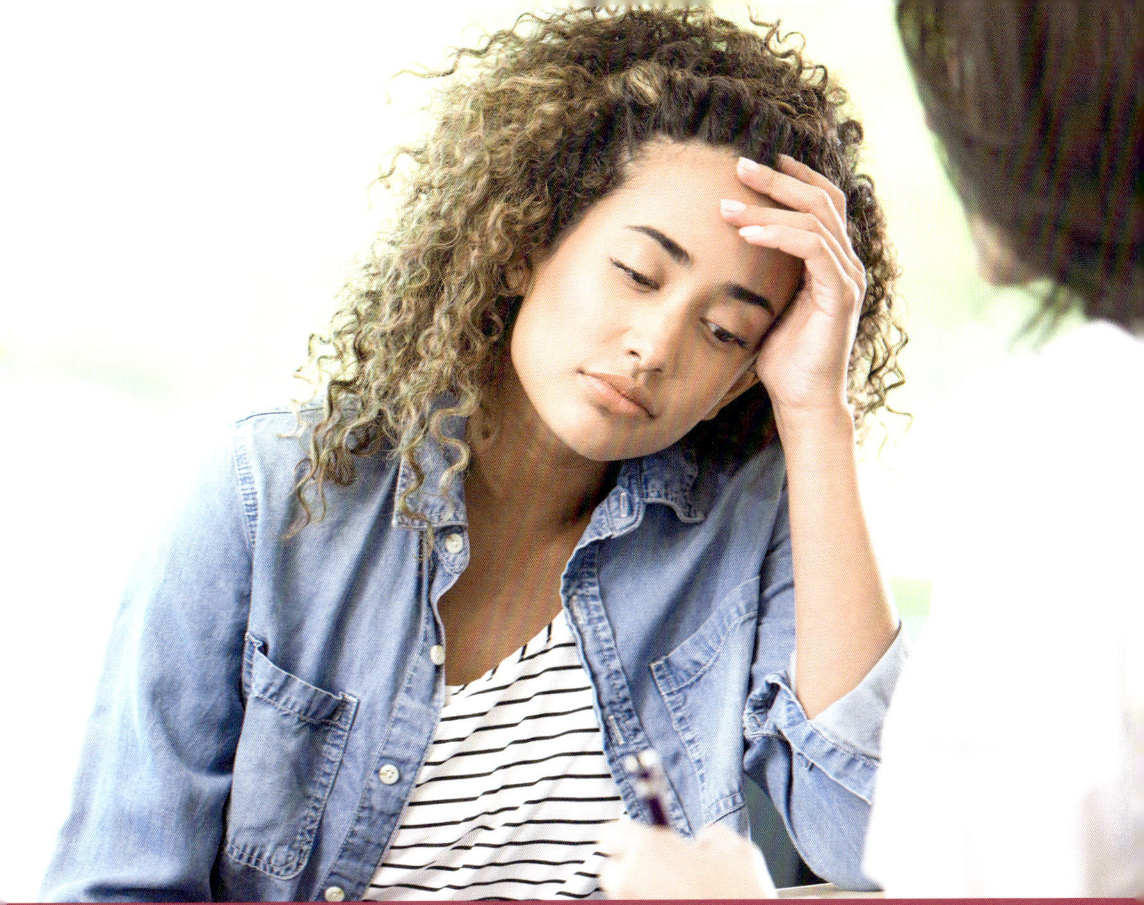

***Stigma can make it harder to talk about eating disorders.***

Stigma causes people with eating disorders to feel ashamed. They may keep their eating behaviors a secret. This can have a serious effect. Stigma prevents people from getting the help they need.

People with eating disorders may be afraid that others will judge them. Dietitian Tammy Beasley spoke about eating disorders and stigma. "An eating disorder feeds on silence. And silence feeds on shame," she said. "Tell someone you trust that you are not okay and that your relationship with your food and body is out of control."[6]

### WEIGHT STIGMA

There is a stigma toward weight in today's society. People feel pressure to match beauty standards. They may fear judgment from others. This can lead to problems with body image. It can also lead to depression. These pressures may lead to behaviors such as binge eating.

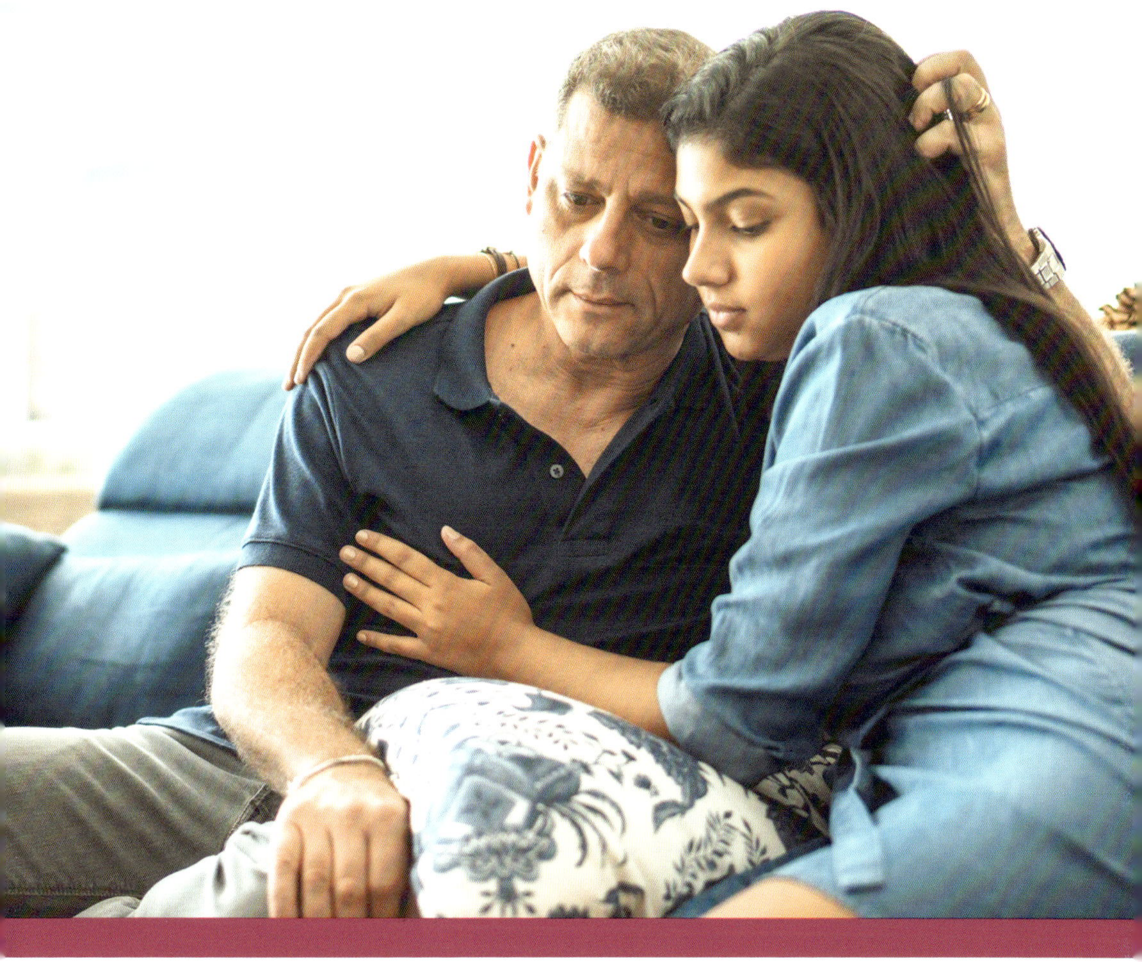

*It can be difficult to see a loved one struggle with an eating disorder.*

## DAILY LIFE AND EATING BEHAVIORS

Eating disorders affect everyday life. People with eating disorders may have a hard time concentrating. This can lead to poor performance in school or at work. Eating disorders can cause someone to avoid friends and family. People with eating disorders may get upset easily.

People suffering from anorexia are focused on weight loss. It interferes with their daily lives. They are constantly thinking about food and weight. They may refuse to

### FASTING FOR RELIGION

Some religions have rituals that ask followers to fast. Catholic people fast on certain days leading up to Easter. Muslim people fast during Ramadan. They do not eat food during the daytime for the entire holy month. These times can be challenging for people with eating disorders. Fasting can lead to eating behaviors that worsen their illnesses.

eat in front of others. They may skip meals or throw the food away.

People with anorexia lose extreme amounts of weight. Children and teens may be much smaller than their peers. It can be very concerning to friends and family members. People with anorexia do not feel thin. They do not understand the severity of their weight loss. They may wear baggy clothes to hide their bodies. They may resist efforts to gain healthy weight.

Someone who binge eats may insist on eating alone. Household members may notice that large amounts of food disappear quickly. They might find numerous empty food containers in the trash. People who binge eat may also hide food in strange places.

## HEALTH CHALLENGES

Eating disorders can lead to other health challenges. People with eating disorders do not take in a healthy amount of nutrients. This puts a lot of stress on the body.

People with anorexia eat too little. They do not get enough energy from food. A person with the disorder may get tired and cold easily. The starvation also affects a person's heart. The heart becomes weak.

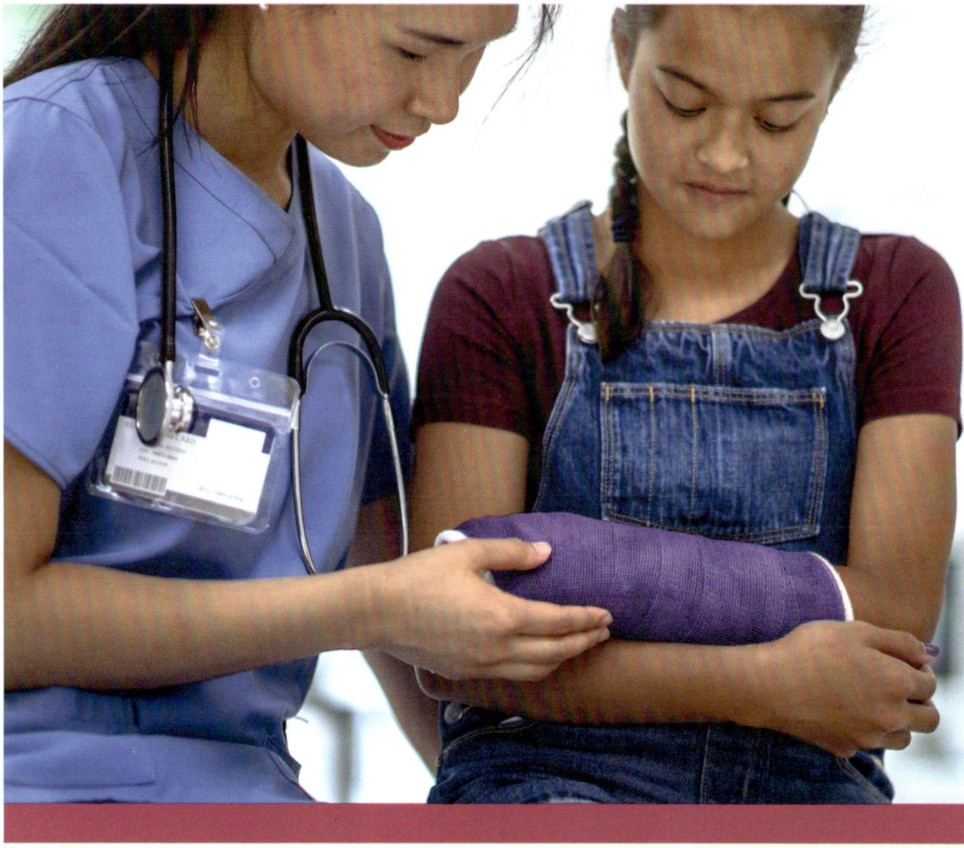

***People with anorexia may be at risk for broken bones due to poor nutrition.***

It has difficulty pumping blood throughout the body. People with anorexia can be at great risk for heart failure.

People with ARFID face similar health challenges. They may have heart problems.

They may have issues with digestion. Their bones weaken from lack of nutrients.

Bulimia hurts a person's health in other ways. Frequent vomiting exposes a person's teeth to stomach acid. The acid can break down teeth over time. It also damages taste receptors. This leads to decreased sensitivity to taste. People without the disorder may get tired of a taste while eating a meal. This is a signal that they are becoming full. People with bulimia do not tire of a taste as quickly. They may not recognize when they are full. This can cause problems with eating habits.

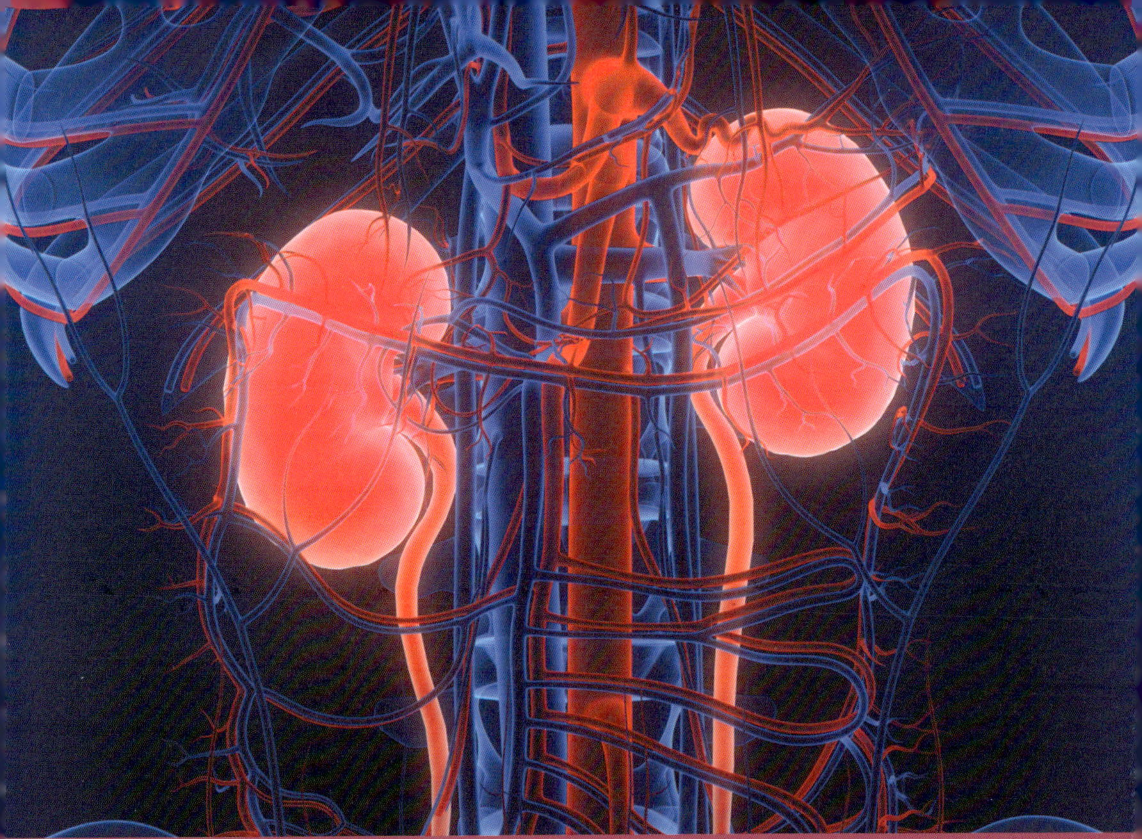

*Bulimia can damage a person's kidneys.*

Purging behaviors can lead to dehydration. This can cause heart issues. It also damages the kidneys. This can be serious. Toxins can build up in the bloodstream. A person with bulimia may need to have a kidney transplant.

Binge eating may affect hormones related to appetite. Some hormones signal that the body is full. They make people feel less hungry. People who binge eat have abnormal levels of these hormones. They still feel hungry after eating. This can lead to more binge eating. Binge eating may also make hormone imbalances more extreme.

Some people with binge eating disorder gain weight from continual overeating. Over time this disease can also lead to serious health problems. People with binge eating disorder often develop high blood pressure. They are also at risk for heart disease.

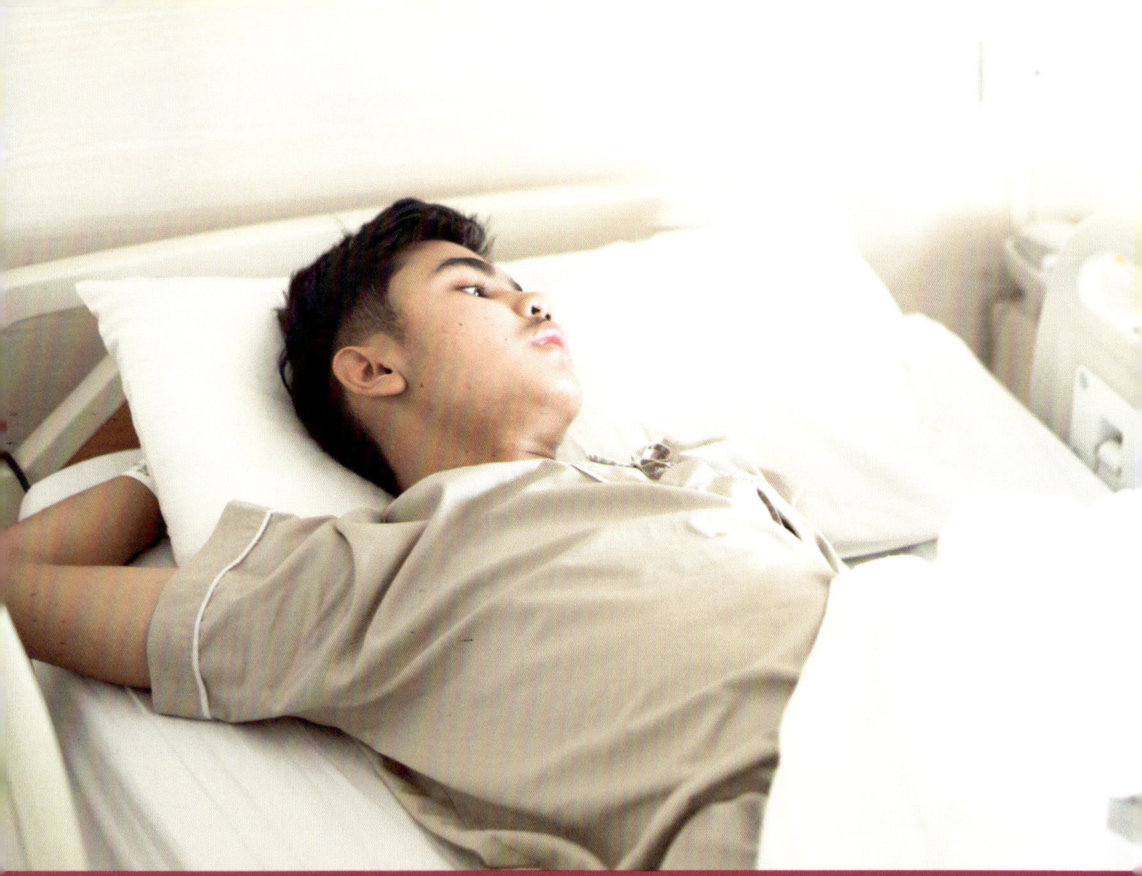

***Eating disorders can have a severe effect on health.***

Having an eating disorder can be dangerous. Not seeking help for it can be deadly. More people die from these diseases each year than any other mental illness.

CHAPTER FOUR

# TREATING EATING DISORDERS

The first step in recovery is asking for help. Someone with an eating disorder can talk to a family doctor. Doctors can perform an initial exam. Doctors rule out other causes for the behaviors. For example, a lack of appetite can be a sign of many other illnesses. Doctors can also

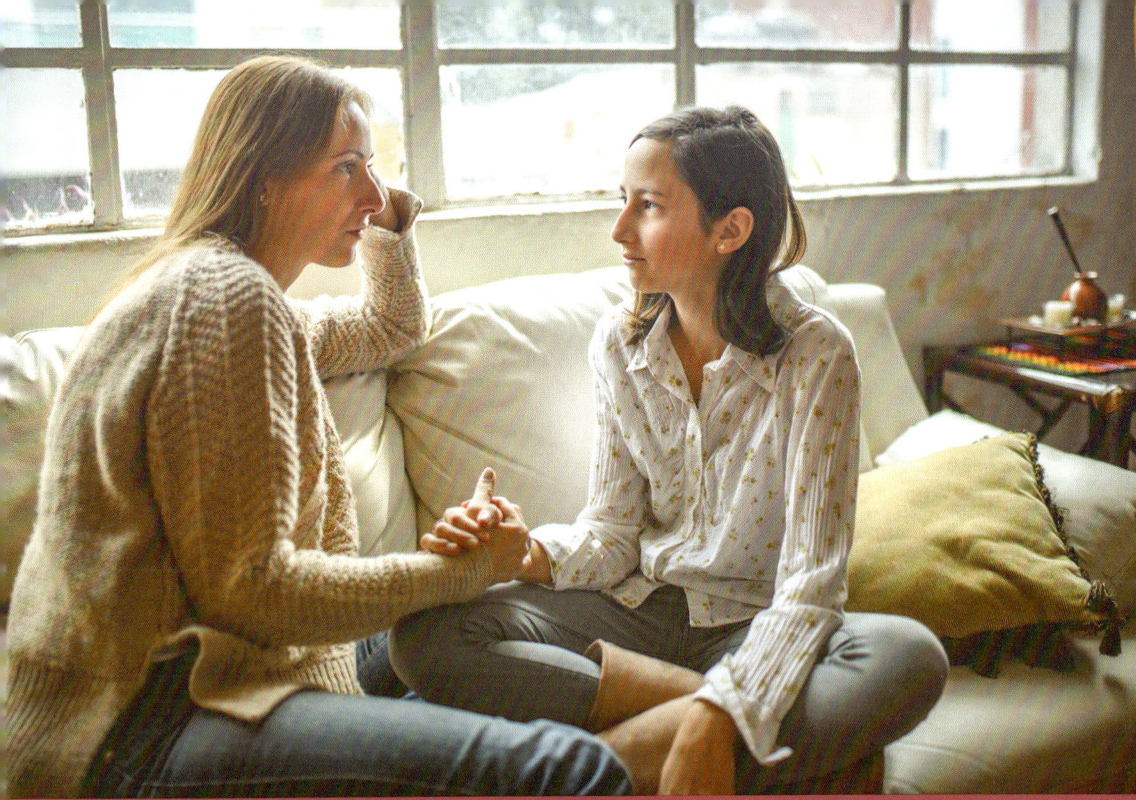

***It can be difficult to talk about an eating disorder and ask for help.***

treat health issues that are caused by the potential eating disorder.

Treatment often begins with psychotherapy. Patients meet with a therapist. They discuss thoughts, feelings, and behaviors that are linked to the eating disorder. Cognitive behavioral therapy (CBT) is a common form of psychotherapy. A therapist may help patients understand their thoughts about food and appearance. CBT helps patients recognize negative thought patterns. Patients learn to change their eating behaviors.

Some patients benefit from group therapy. A therapist leads the patients. People with eating disorders share their experiences with one another. Talking to other people with similar experiences can help patients feel less alone. Group

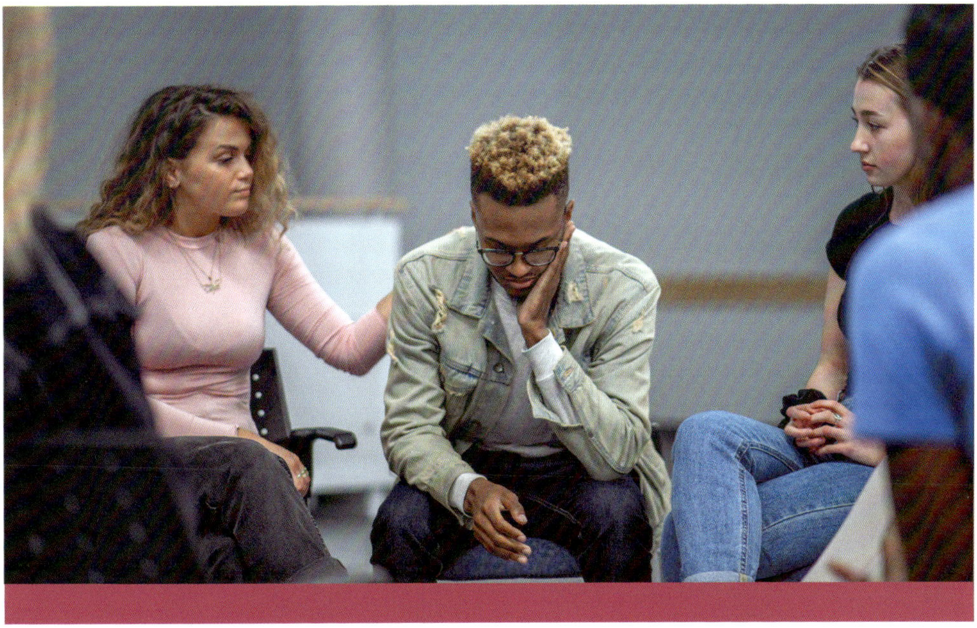

***People with eating disorders may talk about coping strategies during group therapy.***

therapy can also reduce the stigma of eating disorders.

Family-based treatment is another option. Family members may want to learn how to best support a loved one. A therapist offers guidance during this treatment. Family members learn ways to reduce stress. This can help improve eating behaviors.

Many patients can live at home while receiving treatment. But sometimes a hospital stay becomes necessary. This can be discouraging for some patients. But it can also save lives. They can receive constant care from medical professionals. They can focus on recovery away from other stresses. Counselor Jacquelyn Ekern explained, “It may be helpful for the sufferer to consider that taking one step back (into more intensive treatment) will likely launch

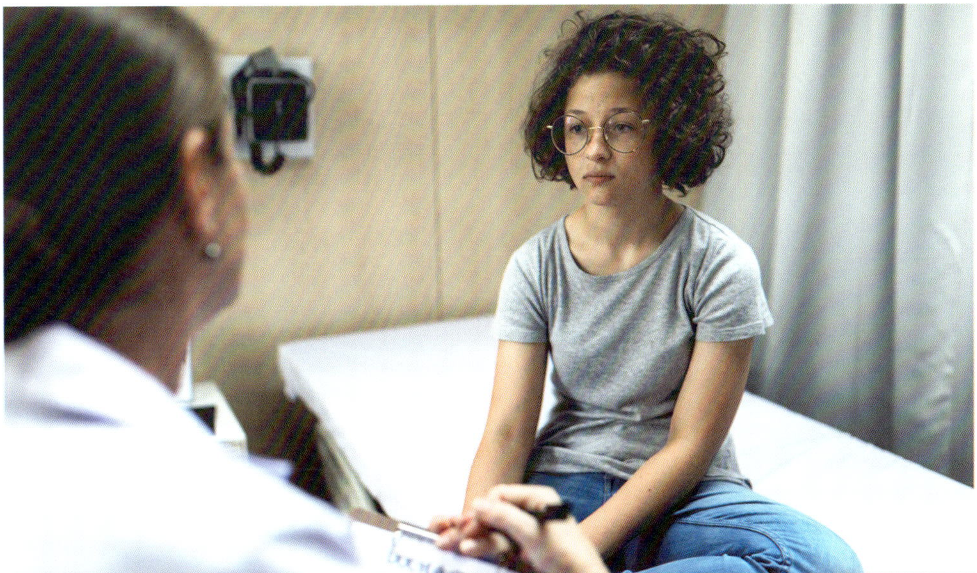

***Regular checkups help ensure that a person with an eating disorder is getting necessary nutrients.***

them two steps forward (greater recovery and health)."[7]

## NUTRITION EDUCATION

Learning about nutrition is a big part of treating an eating disorder. A dietitian teaches patients how to maintain their weight within a healthy range. Patients learn about different types of food. They learn how food helps the body. They also learn about how disordered eating harms their health. Recovering from an eating disorder can be a long and challenging process. It takes time to form healthy habits. Having a nutrition plan in place can be helpful. A nutrition plan can provide structure for eating habits.

Dietitians can help patients with meal planning. They help set up a routine for healthy eating. Patients are typically encouraged to eat three meals a day as well as two or three snacks. Some patients are also taught how to avoid dieting or binge eating. A dietitian can help address other health concerns as well.

Elizabeth Jarrard is a dietitian who works with patients with eating disorders. She works to change her patients' relationships with food. "I work with my clients to remove

## COMPLEMENTARY THERAPIES

**Some patients with eating disorders use complementary therapies. Some examples include relaxation techniques and yoga. These cannot replace psychotherapy and nutrition education. But they can provide benefits when paired with proven treatments.**

the shame, fear, and guilt associated with food, and bring them into a healthier relationship with both food and their bodies."[8]

## MEDICATIONS AND NEW TREATMENTS

Scientists are developing new treatments for eating disorders. They research whether medication can help. Many patients with eating disorders also have anxiety or depression. Doctors may prescribe drugs to treat these conditions.

Some bulimia patients have improved after taking Prozac. This drug is usually used to treat depression. The Food and

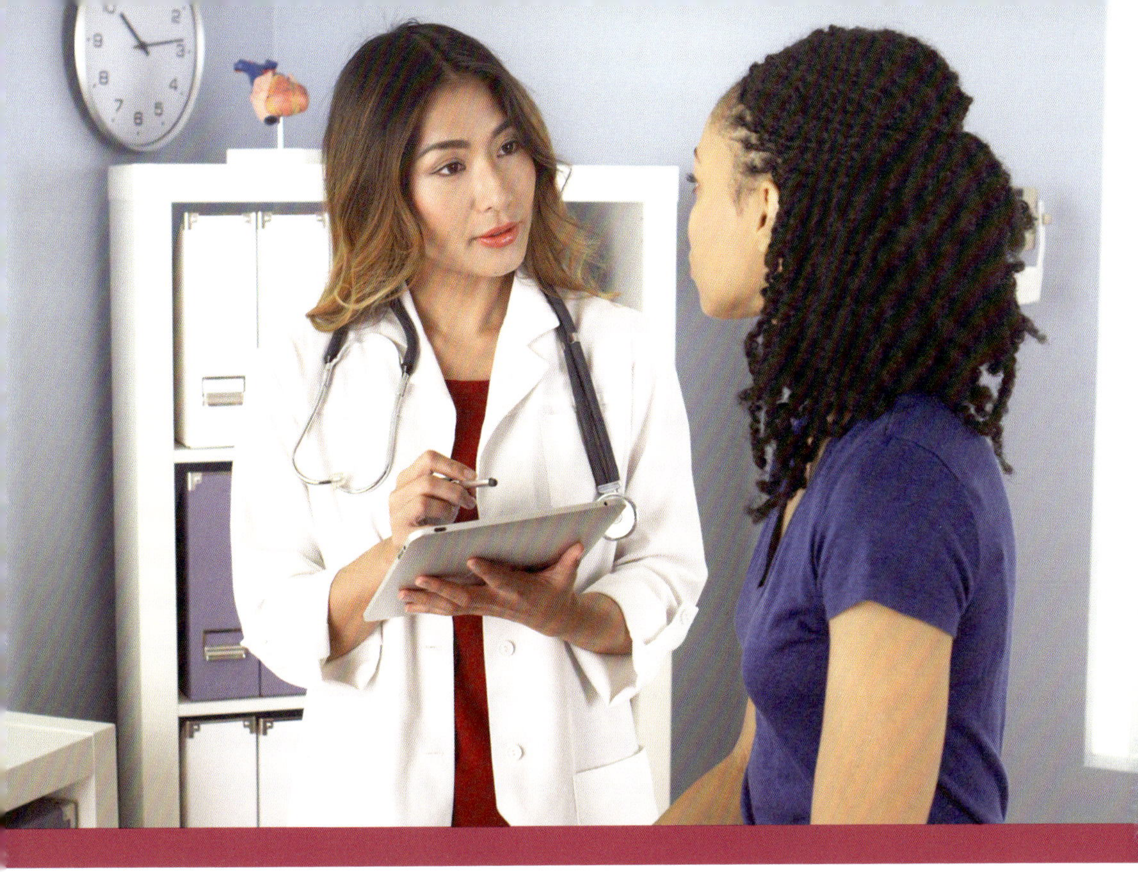

***Medication can be used to supplement treatments for some eating disorders.***

Drug Administration (FDA) approved Prozac to treat bulimia in 1996. It is the only medicine approved to treat the disorder.

The FDA approved Vyvanse to treat binge eating disorder in 2015. This drug was first used to treat attention deficit hyperactivity disorder. But it can also reduce binge eating. Vyvanse can cause severe side effects. It can cause changes in mood. It can worsen heart conditions. Doctors must make sure a patient is healthy enough to take Vyvanse.

Each patient's treatment plan and progress are different. People with eating disorders can learn to manage their symptoms. And treatment can improve their long-term health.

A young woman named Asha began her recovery in a hospital. She learned to take life one day at a time. "I never thought I could be free from my eating disorder, and I have never worked so hard in my life to find that freedom," she wrote. "But it was worth it! Every single day of my recovery journey has been a blessing."[9]

### LAURIE HERNANDEZ

Gymnast Laurie Hernandez has spoken about having bulimia. She struggled with bingeing and purging before the 2016 Olympic Games. After seeking help, Hernandez put a lot of work into her recovery. She now looks at her body very differently than before. She said, "When I was sixteen, the goal was to lose weight, look good, and fit in with the other girls. Now I want to be strong and be able to rely on my body."

*Quoted in Rachel Hosie, "Olympic Gymnast Laurie Hernandez Overcame Years of Binge-Eating and Purging to Focus on Being Strong, Not Skinny,"* Insider, *July 7, 2021. www.insider.com*

# GLOSSARY

**calories**

units of measuring how much energy a food provides

**compulsive**

relating to a strong urge or need

**fasting**

eating little or nothing at all for a period of time

**hormone**

a chemical produced in the body that influences body and brain functions

**laxatives**

medications that cause bowel movements

**psychiatrist**

a doctor who diagnoses and treats mental health conditions

**stereotypes**

oversimplified beliefs about a group of people

**stigma**

a societal attitude about something that creates shame around it and makes people feel embarrassed to be associated with it

# SOURCE NOTES


## CHAPTER ONE: THE HISTORY OF EATING DISORDERS

1. James Greenblatt, "Malorexia: Anorexia Nervosa Redefined," *Psychiatry Redefined*, July 1, 2019. www.psychiatryredefined.org.

2. Quoted in Steffi Lee, "Eating Disorder Survivor Pushes for More Treatment Help," *CBS Iowa*, May 19, 2016. https://cbs2iowa.com.

## CHAPTER TWO: NOTABLE EATING DISORDERS

3. Quoted in Elamin Abdelmahmoud, "This Is What It's Like for Men with Eating Disorders," *Buzzfeed News*, February 6, 2021. www.buzzfeednews.com.

4. Quoted in Rebecca Adams and Eva Hill, "My Struggle with Binge-Eating Disorder," *HuffPost*, December 6, 2017. www.huffpost.com.

## CHAPTER THREE: EATING DISORDERS AND EVERYDAY LIFE

5. Emily T. Troscianko, "Anorexia and Friendship," *Psychology Today*, October 1, 2019. www.psychologytoday.com.

6. Quoted in "Three Experts on the Stigma of Eating Disorders," *Future of Personal Health*, May 7, 2019. www.futureofpersonalhealth.com.

## CHAPTER FOUR: TREATING EATING DISORDERS

7. Jacquelyn Ekern, "How to Determine If Inpatient or Residential Anorexia Treatment Is Necessary?" *Eating Disorder Hope*, January 1, 2015. www.eatingdisorderhope.com.

8. Quoted in "Eating Disorders from the Perspective of a Dietitian: Interview with Elizabeth Jarrard, RD," *Mended Wing Counseling*, n.d. https://mendedwingcounseling.com.

9. Quoted in "What Is Diabulimia?" *Health Partners*, 2022. www.healthpartners.com.

# FOR FURTHER RESEARCH


## BOOKS

Renae Gilles, *Understanding Eating Disorders*. Ann Arbor, MI: Cherry Lake Publishing, 2020.

Hilary W. Poole, *Eating Disorders*. New York: Weigl, 2018.

Kristin Thiel, *Dealing with Eating Disorders*. New York: Cavendish Square, 2020.

## INTERNET SOURCES

Erika Edwards, "Pandemic Created 'Perfect Storm' for Eating Disorders in Teens," *NBC News*, May 24, 2021. www.nbcnews.com.

Kalina Newman, "Eating Disorder Content on Tik-Tok Can Be Both Helpful and Harmful," *Teen Vogue*, July 28, 2020. www.teenvogue.com.

Kara Wahlgren, "8 Dangerous Myths About Eating Disorders That Need to Be Debunked," *Seventeen*, February 26, 2018. www.seventeen.com.

## WEBSITES

### Eating Disorder Hope
**www.eatingdisorderhope.com**

Eating Disorder Hope was founded in 2005. The organization offers information and support to people with eating disorders.

### National Association of Anorexia Nervosa and Associated Disorders (ANAD)
**https://anad.org**

ANAD is a nonprofit organization that offers peer support to people with eating disorders. The volunteers have struggled with eating disorders themselves.

### National Eating Disorders Association (NEDA)
**www.nationaleatingdisorders.org**

NEDA is the largest nonprofit organization for people affected by eating disorders. It helps individuals and families get the help they need.

# INDEX

# IMAGE CREDITS

Cover: © Goran 13/iStockphoto
5: © Enes Evren/iStockphoto
7: © Wavebreak Media/ Shutterstock Images
9: © Raw Pixel/Shutterstock Images
11: © Drazen Zigic/iStockphoto
13: © Monkey Business Images/ iStockphoto
15: © bubutu/Shutterstock Images
16: Jean Honoré Fragonard/ Metropolitan Museum of Art
19: © SDI Productions/iStockphoto
23: © kali 9/iStockphoto
27: © Bear Fotos/Shutterstock Images
29: © Red Line Editorial
31: © Cocopelli/Shutterstock Images
33: © Raw Pixel/Shutterstock Images
36: © Renee Clancy/ Shutterstock Images
38: © Tirachard/iStockphoto
40: © Cheap Books/ Shutterstock Images
42: © By Muratdeniz/iStockphoto
45: © Mikolette/iStockphoto
47: © Amazing Mikael/iStockphoto
48: © Daisy Daisy/Shutterstock Images
51: © SDI Productions/iStockphoto
53: © Pollyana Ventura/iStockphoto
57: © Fat Camera/iStockphoto
59: © Magic mine/Shutterstock Images
61: © Komsan Loonprom/ Shutterstock Images
63: © M Studio Images/iStockphoto
65: © Fat Camera/iStockphoto
67: © Raw Pixel/iStockphoto
71: © Rocketclips, Inc./ Shutterstock Images

# ABOUT THE AUTHOR

Tammy Gagne has written dozens of books for both adults and children. Some of her recent books have covered media literacy and social justice. She lives in northern New England with her husband and son.